Dangerous Love

Divorce Your Diet and Learn How to Eat Healthy, Get More Energy and Lose Weight Permanently.

Ilan Halfon

Printed in Canada and the United States

Edited by Conclusio Inc., Toronto, Canada

First Printing, 2011
Second Printing, 2014

ISBN-13: 978-1499396003
ISBN-10: 1499396007

Preston Squire Publishing
261 Oakwood Ave
York, ON, M6E 2V3

Acknowledgements

One thing that I love and have learned to appreciate is the people and teachers that have come my way. Thanks to their influence, this book has become a reality for me.

In particular, I would like to say thank you to:

Irad Carpel for being everything I could have wished for.

Anita, Tony, Robyn, Mindy, Carol, Raja, Martin, Milton, Marissa, Danny, Nickol, Lisa, Maya, Marcie, Sophie, Mara, Heela, Gidon, Sharon, Dina, Mohamed, Sarita, Tammy, Jessica, Dafna, Valerie, Rachel, Aviva, and finally, our dog Nikita, and cat Sally.

There are so many more individuals that I am grateful for, and two without whom I would not be here at all.

Thank you Mom and Dad for the amazing family you have given me.

I LOVE YOU!

Preface

So, why am I writing this book?

When I initially started FitMe Training Professional Trainers, I was looking for a way to help people, aside from my clients. In trying to reach out to the wider community, I decided to write an article for a Toronto magazine.

When I gave the article to some of my clients and friends to review, many of them commented that I should take the concept and turn it into a book.

Writing a book was and still is a very big dream for me. I had tried many times before to write one, but was never sure where to begin and, after several false starts, I shelved the idea.

As I continued to work with my clients, I noticed that in my motivational talks I would often respond to what my client had said with, "One of my other clients is facing the exact same challenge."

Most of us, if not all of us, face similar challenges in our lives. Some of us feel guilty about it and some of us don't, but I think it is safe to say that all of us would like to change our lives for the better, wherever possible.

This inspired me to take some of my favourite life memories and lessons (most of which, to my surprise, involved my clients) and compile them into this book, which has been a privilege for me to write. This book is a little collection of advice I've given my clients (or learned from them), so if you are a reader who has the desire and strength of will to make a change in your life—to be better, healthier, and to achieve the body you've dreamt of—then all you need to do is follow and practice what you read here.

FitMe Training is not just about training for a healthier body. Anyone who knows me will agree that I believe in keeping things in the proper perspective. So what is FitMe all about? FitMe is about setting out on a life journey to a healthier lifestyle for yourself and for those close to you.

All the best, with love,

Ilan

We want to thank you for purchasing FitMe Everywhere's book: Dangerous Love

As a special Thank You we have created Four Bonus Features for you to download, absolutely FREE, from our Facebook Page at: www.fb.com/FitMeTraining

Please LIKE the page so you can continue to receive tips, encouragement and other bonus items in future.

Your Bonus Gifts provide insights on:

1. Great sources of plant-based nutrition
2. Learn about the benefits of Cleansing
3. Why I love Yoga (and you will too)
4. 1500 calorie menu

75% OFF BONUS OFFER

Post a picture of your favorite unhealthy food or a picture of your copy of the Dangerous Love book/ebook with #mydangerouslove on your Facebook page and receive a LIVE nutritional consultation with author and fitness expert Ilan Halfon for only $25 (a $100 value).

Table of Contents

FitMe to Say "Bye-Bye Sugar"

In life, we all face times when we have big choices to make, such as "Should I stay in the relationship I'm currently in, or should I end it and make a commitment to a new one?" I trust that by the end of this journey, you would have made a decision of your own, a choice by which you will stand.

I now see my former pattern of decision-making for what it was—a set of negative habits that created an abusive relationship. A relationship, as I see it, is a collection of habits, both good and bad. This is true of almost any relationship once a certain amount of time has passed. But in this instance, I am talking about the biggest relationship of all, one you cannot live without; the one that even before you are born, already has a huge impact on your being.

For me, when it came to choosing one thing or another, I had to make the decision to hit rewind on the relationship I had with my body (yes, we all have a relationship with our bodies). Why am I talking about having a relationship with my body? Because it was that mindset that helped me to get healthy. Understanding that I have a relationship with my body has helped me to make a huge transformation in my entire being. Once I began to think about my body in this new way, it became a pivotal turning point. I learned to stop taking my body for granted and, when presented with choices, I began to make decisions in a new way.

I used to choose my "dates" (I refer to them as dates because this analogy helps me to better understand my choices prior to making any decision) without using any common sense. I did not think about the effect that my next "date" would have on me. I did not even stop to consider, "Who am I about to date?" Looking back, I can say that it was just about sex. Sex. Sex. Sex. Sorry if I offend anyone, but I am trying to make a point about how bad my relationship with my body really was.

I used to think that whoever I dated had some kind of irresistible power over me, that they could win me over by tantalizing me with their body or with the enticing scent of their own unique perfume. While my eyes were tempted, it was mainly their perfume, that special scent that would make me lose control over my entire being. It was their aroma that I couldn't resist, the whiff of freshness, that fragrance that you smell only in the morning. While faced with these huge temptations, I tried to make the right decisions. As I took in their amazing scent I was supposed to say, "No, no thanks."

The worst part was that even when they couldn't tempt me with their smell, they would still entice me with the shape of their bodies. Oh gosh, the way they looked! They would wear all these beautiful colours, and some of them were decorated in strong reds, whites, greens, and yellows (my favourites). You name it, they were wearing it. Anyone who knows me knows how easy it is to tempt me with colour. The smells were right there, the colours were right there, so making the right choice was something that I could not have started doing, until I began to understand my relationship behaviour. Now what used to look very sexy to me is not even worth a second glance.

Up until this point, I haven't given my sexy former dates a name, but what I am really talking about is 'sexy breads,' and 'sexy baked goods' (more like baked 'bads').

It was these supposedly 'sexy' carbs and SUGAR ⍰ to which I was addicted. There it is, I've said it! I was addicted to 'dating' sugar.

I remember how I used to think about my next date with sugar even when I was currently on a date. I remember thinking about our weekends together, thinking about our nights. I was all over the place in my mind.

Sugar, sugar, and more sugar.

The worst part about being in a relationship with sugar is that it has its way of getting into you through all types of dressings, smells, colours, and, to hell with it, I might as well say it now, it can even get to you in a salty way. Yes, a salty way, in items that are a version of sugar. Smell, shape, colour, you name it; the sugar tempted me in a way that only sugar can. It even tempted me in the form of a bag of chips.

One of my many experiences started like this: I was walking down the street with no cravings whatsoever for anything. You know the feeling, the times when you just walk down the street knowing where you need to be and what time you need to be there. This was one of those moments for me. I was on the way to a business meeting and as I was walking, I passed a small bakery or a Starbucks. All of a sudden it hit me, that aroma again. That freshness that I thought you could only smell in the morning. The second it went through my system, just after the first breath, even before I had realized it, I was already paying for one large muffin and a double-sized latte. In the same breath as my order, I would say, "Oh, and please be sure to make my latte sugar-free" (as if the muffin contained only protein and air calories). At this point I didn't even have a choice when it came to my actions. I am talking about an out-of-control sugar addiction.

We all have stories like this one in our past. We all get those cravings almost every day of our lives. We all go on 'dates.' We are all in a relationship in one way or another with sugar, salt, and just about any type of habit that prevents us from having a successful relationship with our bodies.

This chapter is about helping us all to understand that what we eat, the way we eat, and how much we eat, can either lead us to be in an abusive relationship or to have one of the most beautiful relationships ever between ourselves and our bodies.

So, you may ask, "What changed?" How did I manage to break the cycle of dating my ex-lover? Well, I will say that I have met a new date and have formed dating habits of a different style. I chose not to be the slut of sugar, and I chose not to be the person bitten by the sugar bully.

I choose to take a stand. I choose to take full responsibility for my relationship. Please don't get me wrong, I am still dating sugar, but now I have dressed it with a different smell and have given it different shapes. I have divorced the old sugar and now I have added so many other colours into our relationship that it has become an everlasting love story.

I went in a whole new direction, a way of making choices that are free of emotion. Now, I spread all my options out in front of me and consider them before making my decision.

And let me tell you, if I can make that change, then so can anyone. How? If you wish to know, then you have already found yourself in the right place, with the right book in your hands.

FitMe to Divorce My Ex

So what happened that caused me to contemplate divorcing my ex? The best way to continue this story is to pick up where I left off in the last chapter.

As I made my way to that business meeting, you will recall that I had found myself in line for a large muffin and a non-fat, sugar-free latte. In that same coffee and bakery shop was a very annoying person just ahead of me in the line. I already knew what I wanted to order and wished that he did too, but instead he was asking the person behind the counter question after question about this item and that item. Now, I was more than a little beat and in a rush. "Grrr," I bristled. "Why, why, why did he have to ask so many questions? Why the hell couldn't he just order what he wanted and move on?" It's just another snack, and he was making me late for my meeting.

Please allow me to tell you that this moment could not have gotten any better than that. After getting what I wanted, I headed to my meeting. I always like to be early to my meetings, but thanks to this person I thought I might be late.

As I walked, I ate my muffin and sipped my non-fat, sugar-free latte. I was caught up in my own illusion that it was okay to have this type of latte, not considering the fact that this latte equaled half of my lunch. You might have your eyes wide open, but you read right. This non-fat, sugar-free latte contained almost half of the calorie value of my lunch that day. Not that I really make a habit of counting calories, but I want to make a point here.

As I was walking out of the coffee shop, I saw, through the window, the same annoying man-of-many-questions sitting and eating his order. It just annoyed me even more to see that, after all of the questions he had asked, he still hadn't ordered coffee, or a muffin, or any of the baked goods that one normally has with coffee.

At the end of the day it looked like he had chosen a large smoothie or maybe some odd-coloured iced coffee. Whatever he was drinking, it looked good, but I still could not figure out why he had needed to ask so many questions.

After a short five minute walk, I had reached my destination. I didn't know what the person I was supposed to meet looked like, so we had agreed that he would call me on my cell phone once he arrived at the place.

As I was waiting, my cell phone began to ring, and as I reached for it, I saw that annoying guy walking up with his cell phone in hand. He was looking around to check whose phone would ring, but I was already approaching him to say "Hello." In my mind, I already knew that he had lost any points he might have possibly won with me. After seeing him in the coffee shop, I expected he would be a boring person, the kind who has no idea what he wants.

As we sat down, it was very difficult for me to start the meeting without sharing my thoughts about his behaviour in the coffee shop moments before. I told him that I had been right behind him in the line, and though I couldn't exactly hear what he had been asking, it sounded like way too many questions. He only had to order a coffee and a snack, but he was making it far too complicated. I finished my short story by telling him that he looked like one of those people who don't know what they want. "I know it may sound a bit rude, but don't you think that holding up the line on a busy morning at a coffee shop is a bit rude?"

"Well," he said, "you know, you might be right. Maybe I don't really know what I want. However, the thing is, it's not that I don't know what I want. I know exactly what I want. The questions help me to make the right choice so that I will choose what I *need*." He continued to tell me that most people just follow what they want and, in most cases, fall into the trap of making the wrong choices for themselves because they wish to satisfy a craving for a moment of pleasure.

He explained to me that as he asked all those questions, which I had found so annoying, he was creating a full "spreadsheet" of all the choices he could make. He explored his options so that he could choose what he needed. He told me that now what he eats, for the most part, is also what he wants. He used to go into a coffee shop and let his eyes and nose do the choosing for him, and then he would feel like crap for the rest of the day. He had since learned that what he wanted and what he needed, were not always the same thing. Then he explained to me what he meant when he said "spreadsheet."

You see, for this man, there were a few things that he would do whatever he could to avoid, notably sugar and dairy. Those two were always labeled in his mind as "stay away," not because they were forbidden due to some health concern, but because he made a choice to stay away from them.

If he saw something that appealed to his eyes, all he needed to do was think about whether it contained any of the things on the "stay away" list that he had on the spreadsheet in his mind.

That was the point of all the questions he was asking. They were actually all variations of the same question: "Does this product contain any of the ingredients I have on my stay away list?" You see, most people who are trying to eat healthy wouldn't eat chocolate cake, but they might have cheese cake. For this man it was easy, neither of them was an option.

"So if it doesn't contain any of the items on your stay away list, will you have it?" I asked.

It turned out that it was a bit more complicated to explain. For the most part, he would start asking questions to understand the source of whatever it was that he was about to consume. "But," I said to him, "you ended up having something that looked like a smoothie. As far as I know smoothies have loads of sugar, don't they?" He told me that I was absolutely right; smoothies do have loads of sugar. However, his was water-based, with fruit and veggies combined (spinach, celery, and green apple). Once he had all his options laid out in front of him, choosing one or another, or maybe even none, became very easy for him. He told me that he had gone to that place because he needed a snack before meeting me, as he was running a bit behind and had skipped taking his snack with him from home. And then he asked me why I had gone into the coffee shop.

That was exactly what snapped me out of it. The small question he ended with was what changed everything for me and became the genesis for this book about starting the journey to a better, healthier life.

FitMe Makes the Needs Into Wants

Why is it so difficult for most people to pursue what it is that they need? How is it that when it comes to the "I need to do..." stuff, it takes us such a long time to get around to it, even though we know it needs to be done? Or, even more often than that, people begin to take positive action only to give it up shortly afterwards. They will encounter a moment when things aren't going smoothly or coming easily, and they think to themselves, "Ok, maybe I don't really need to do this, maybe my body is fine just the way it is." Admittedly, you and your body might be fine just the way you are, but the point is not whether or not you are alright the way you are, the point is, why is it that you gave up and turned around on your dream of being slimmer, healthier, stronger or more fit (or whatever it is that you are aiming to achieve)?

Well, I can't answer that question on behalf of all people, but I can speak for myself. I can tell you that for me, as an ex-fat person, that I used all the excuses in the world to others, but most of all to myself. Excuses like having big bones or being too tall for my age. The excuses would go on and on. Now I know that a healthy weight is mainly a matter of practice. If I had the tools then that I have today, it would have been faster for me to lose all that weight.

When I say that it was a matter of practice, I mean that it was and still is a process, a process of understanding that it isn't about losing 60 pounds, or getting a six-pack and the most toned body I can manage. It isn't about starving myself and it isn't about being skinny. It is about being in control of my body, it is about being aware of everything that I eat, and it is about finding balance with my health. There it is, the tagline of all my preaching—be in balance with your health.

Whenever I thought about making a change, like going on a diet, it was that dream of being skinny with a toned body that gave me the full motivation I needed to take the first step when I was 230 pounds.

Unfortunately, by the third step I would have already given up. For the most part, the reason for my failure was mainly because I was not thinking or planning ahead in my mind. I didn't prepare myself for the moments, which used to come pretty often, where I would feel tempted to fall back into my old habits. I didn't plan how I would act when things became hard or when there was temptation right in front of me. I didn't consider what would happen once my eating habits became less colourful on a diet. I used to hate the word "diet." If you break it into two words you get DIE EAT. That was the feeling I used to get, that I would die if I ate like I am supposed to eat on a diet. Today, I have come to the understanding that a diet is just another word for lifestyle, and that each and every one of us creates our own lifestyle. So now I have made that one word into four words:

Do

I

Eat

That?

This takes me back to the spreadsheet we talked about in the previous chapter. Looking back from where I am today, the spreadsheet could have made things so much easier for me, since this is one of the best tools when choosing the right path and seeing what needs to be done. As I mentioned before, we often choose what we want instead of what we need.

Very often I ask my clients, "Why did you make that unhealthy choice? Don't you know that you will pay the price by having to workout so much harder or by cutting out snacks for the coming 3–4 days?" And as often as I ask that question, the answer will be, "I wanted it so much, I couldn't resist it." I WANTED.

What about what you needed? What about the impact of that decision? I also want one million dollars in my bank account really badly. If I wanted to go rob a bank I could, but I would have to pay the price afterwards.

The same thing goes with choosing what you want instead of what you need. You will pay the price of being in your own prison.

For me, as a big dreamer (a really big dreamer), I always tell my clients, "You must visualize yourself exactly where you wish to be. You must see yourself like you have already made it to your destination. You must place your body, mind, and spirit wherever it is that you want to go. However, and this is a big however, you must be logical as well. You must find balance between your vision and the present moment. You need to be able to distinguish between the two. It is all about the path that you are choosing to walk on, and it is about understanding the process that you must follow in order to reach that vision. You will have to clear the path for yourself, and you have to understand that the road can get hectic, that you might meet turbulence, that you will face lots of temptations, and that you are going to be living your current life at the same time as you are stepping into your new way of living. Choosing the path of FitMe in order to change your needs to wants is all about living your life to the fullest."

For instance, many rich people say that in order to become rich you must think like a rich person. It is not about buying whatever you want whenever you want it; it is about making plans to get what you want and ensuring that your bank account can afford it. It's about giving up your luxurious lifestyle in order to save money so that you can invest in the right places. I am not rich, but I interview lots of wealthy people and I am extremely rich in my own way ☐. The rich people I know tell me that it's about saving money for what you want so that you don't head towards debt, and that if you must take money from your credit, then make sure to replace it. You will be earning more than you will be spending at the end of the day. They often tell me that it is about being patient.

The same thing is true for us when choosing this path of health; we must be patient. It is much easier to gain the weight than it is to say goodbye to a few extra pounds. When you implement this new lifestyle, even if you make a choice that is based on what you want instead of what you need, you know you can always balance things out afterwards.

A healthy person who has an extra portion of sugar or a glass of alcohol, something that they know they would have been better off without, will already be planning ahead. They know that tomorrow or later on that same day they will have to go for a nice long jog or that they will have to cut the sugar out of the following day. You cannot fall into the trap of making one bad decision after another or else you will find that things will snowball and you will end up in an unhealthy loop. So, you have made an unhealthy choice, it's done, now get up and pay the price, keep yourself in motion.

It's about creating a balance in your day-to-day living. It's about understanding that by choosing the path of healthy living, you will learn to make the choices that you need to make versus the ones that you think you want. Choosing what you want is just a way to avoid making a harder choice, and it is also a way of making choices without really thinking about them first.

FitMe to Be a Role Model

You might be thinking to yourself, "Is this guy crazy?" FitMe a role model? Haha...What is he talking about?"

I am talking about the most important thing that we are surrounded by, and that is our loved ones. I am asking you if you can be a role model for them, or if you will be a follower. I remember when I became vegan (don't worry, I am not trying to preach veganism to you here. I just wanted to mention it. For me veganism is not just about avoiding eating animals. For me it is very much a health choice. I used to think that veganism was unhealthy, but then I went into a vegan grocery store and had my first look at vegan cream cheese... but anyways, let me get back to my story) for the first time a major declaration/statement was not easy to get out of my mouth. I didn't come to my partner in life saying, "I am going to go vegan." I actually did my best to keep it as quiet as possible. It was as simple a choice as could be. Once I knew that it was a pure choice that could be reversed anytime, I began to tell myself each and every moment that I live life the way I do by the choices that I make every single day, heck, every single moment.

Being a wellness coach, I often hear the sweetest parents in the world throwing the blame on their kids. They tell me that they cannot have a healthier household because their kids need cookies, they must have French fries, they must have this and they must have that. They see it in school and on TV and the list goes on and on.

Really, I cannot believe that people go so far as to blame their own kids. I can tell you that as a kid who grew up in a full house (a family of six kids) I saw so many brands of fancy things that I wanted, cool shoes, cool clothing, big houses, but did I get them all? Definitely not. For the most part, I didn't get any of them. Don't get me wrong here, my parents are the best in the world, but they worked overly hard for their living and raised six kids with no nanny or whatever luxury most of us are used to having today. They really did it all themselves, so I am not blaming them for not making more of an effort to buy me all of the brands I dreamed of.

I will also say that what these people are telling me about their kids might be absolutely right, and being outside of your family, I don't have the right to doubt it, but you do know yourself better.

Your kids, like any other kids, will look up to their parents. They will do the best they can to act like you, like the little girl who tries on her mother's high heels or the little boy who pretends to be his father. They use us, the adults, as their role models, so although they are the biggest leaders in a house, at the same time they are also the biggest followers.

With that said, what makes you think it will be different with food? What makes you think that choosing to keep a healthier house should depend on waiting for your kids to leave it? Do you want them to grow up having the same fights you are having with your lifestyle? I don't think so.

What I am saying here is that the only place a healthier lifestyle should start is with us. If you are the wife of the house, then please, please, please don't try to force your man or any of the kids in your house to join you. Been there, tried that, didn't work. If you are the man of the house, same thing. The change begins with your own body only. Remember that it is a choice that you are making. You had the time to process things in your mind and to mentally prepare yourself for it, but the people around you have not had that same time, and most likely have not had the chance to argue with themselves about their lifestyle.

By taking the step of diving into the journey of a new lifestyle you will lead them to follow you. You can just make your family the food that you normally do and then cook something healthy for yourself. Let them laugh at you, as that's what normally happens. They will joke around when they see what you are eating, and you can join in when they joke. It will help you to remember that this is a choice you have made for yourself to live a healthier life.

I know it is not that easy to cook for them and cook for yourself, but aren't you always bragging that you are a power multi-tasker? Here is a chance to use it. Besides, cooking and eating healthy is much easier, quicker, and, above all, much cheaper than a regular lifestyle.

We all know that we should worry more about what our kids see than what they hear. Kids will follow your ways. When we were kids, we all wanted to be like our mothers and fathers; we all looked up to and admired them. If you start to show that you are proud of your lifestyle, it will be a process that your entire household will learn to appreciate.

So, where do you begin? How about right here, right now. It is all about remembering that wherever you go and whatever you choose to eat or not to eat your loved ones are with you. At your next meal, with or without your kids, make sure you know what they are going to have and what it is that you are going to have. You should get yourself mentally ready for the small temptation that you might have when your family eats some of the things that you used to love.

In the beginning, I recommend keeping things as simple as possible and not going overboard with your menu. Try to eat similar things from one day to another; let your family get used to what you are eating. Normally, when a new change arrives to a house, it is only fully accepted once it becomes habit. And this is what I am aiming for with this book, to help you change some of your existing habits to brand-new ones. Allow yourself to become the role model that your household can look up to. Allow yourself to live your life to the fullest with the body you dream of. Allow yourself to take the FitMe journey to a whole new level.

Note:

100 grams of almonds equal more than 4 snacks. The cost of 100 grams of almonds is approximately $1.50. The total calorie value is 580 calories. And this is without telling you about all the amazing properties that almonds hold. One large latte with a muffin equals the same amount of calories

but will cost you 3 to 4 times the price and will be consumed in one meal (and by the way that could be a non-fat, sugar-free latte and a whole-wheat muffin.) And you want to tell me that a healthy lifestyle is expensive?

FitMe My Jog Meal

Really? There is something like that? FitMe actually has something that's called a jog meal? Hello, we sure do. Here is how it works.

You know how sometimes on the weekend when you have nothing to do and you are just "vegging out" on your sofa and the only movement your body does besides turning from one side to the other is the walk to the kitchen or to the snack cabinet? I know someone who actually moved their kitchen cabinet to the living room just under the sofa. These days they even design sofas with storage under the arms or legs, anything to help you get comfortable (by the way, remind me to tell you to change that snack cabinet to an almond cabinet, minimizing your snack options and helping you to avoid overeating.) Anyway, back to the sofa and the jog meal.

Once, in a business meeting, I was told that our host had really gone overboard and ordered a fully vegan meal so that I would feel comfortable. He really did his best to get only healthy food and more than just one or two side dishes.

When he saw me eating and really enjoying the meal, he was very happy, until he noticed that I had stopped eating. I avoided a lot of other things that were offered on the table. For me, it was about choosing one or two of the dishes that were offered to us. I had minimized my options to start with. For me, eating and talking business don't go together. As a matter of fact, eating and talking in general don't go together. I am one of those people who can only do one thing at a time. Therefore, all my focus was on being patient while the others finished their meals so that we could start talking some business.

When he noticed me not eating, he was surprised, since he was sure that a personal trainer, among the other things that I do, would need to eat much more. He said that he was used to those trainers or even those muscular guys at buffets eating like there was no tomorrow, and he was sure that I was one of them. When he asked me how come I had stopped eating, it hit me. I had to think for a second to explain myself, and the best thing I could come up with was the FitMe Jog Meal. I told him that for me, every meal is a jog meal, meaning that it is very important to be able to go out for a jog after every meal I have. When I eat, I always bear this in mind. I can tell you that when you eat properly, a small bite can change your whole experience with the meal. Just one more bite and you will either feel satisfied or you will feel full and bloated.

One of my best teachers once said, "You should eat like a king in the morning, a prince at lunch, and a poor man in the evening." That small bite can make a huge difference to every meal, especially the ones you have on the weekend.

He asked me if I was going out for a jog after the meal. I said "Obviously not." Though whoever knows me knows that I love working out. It is still something that I only do five times a week, and except for Saturday, my favourite gym day, when my workouts are an hour and a half, normally my workouts are forty minutes. So, every meal that I have—

breakfast, lunch, dinner or any snack—I am always asking myself if I would be able to go for a jog if I wanted to once I am finished. I eat light enough to keep myself in motion, meaning that I finish my meal satisfied, not full, and not hungry. I have a sensation of feeling light and yet energized that keeps me going throughout my day.

The key point of this chapter is that we should all aim to be in motion. Feeling light after a meal can help you to stay motivated to do other things, because feeling heavy after a meal is the same snowball that can take you all the way back to vegging out.

How can you make that decision? How can that change take place in your life?

After we ask the first question of DIET= Do I Eat This? We will need to ask ourselves another question, maybe even more than one: Should I finish that? Will I feel light enough that I can jog?

I try to be constantly aware of my actions, so instead of talking to others while I eat, I talk to myself, after all it is I who will be carrying my body after each meal, not them.

Tip: Try to stay light with your body. Feeling heavy is an easy thing to avoid. It's called the jog meal.

Thanks for reminding me to explain a bit more about your snack cabinet. Most people keep their snack cabinets full. There will be snacks for each and every member of the family (again, this is where the kids or the partners are to be blamed) and the things that I see in these cabinet—cookies, granola bars, chocolate, you name it, it's there. The whole story of the almond cabinet began when, not so long ago, me and my partner in life moved into our own place. One of my favourite clients came with us to see the place before the renovations, and as the concerned mother that she is (what can I say, she worries about me too much), one of her questions was about the kitchen, as in how will I organize it? When we got to the kitchen, I pointed to the first closet that I saw and immediately said, "This is my almond cabinet."

She was laughing at me so hard, "A whole cabinet just for almonds, you are unbelievable," she said.

You see, it's not about having your kitchen full. I go to the grocery store sometimes three or four times a week, but it takes me maybe ten minutes, since I always know what I need. I get straight to the point, buying exactly what we need, so we save tons of money because we never throw away food that we didn't use. What I am trying to say is that eating is a big part of my day, and I do eat a lot, however it is pretty much the same things that I eat in different shapes and colours.

When it comes to snacking, I keep it as simple as possible, either almonds or fruit. Okay, sometimes both, but either way fruit won't be in my snack cabinet; that is only for the almonds. Some things, regardless of how much we like them, should not be brought into the house.

My partner in life is always saying to me, "As long as I don't see it in the house, I don't crave it." You know what? That is a very smart technique to use.

Tip: Keep your menu simple, colourful, and straight to the point—carbs, proteins, fat, vitamins, minerals. But most important of all, make sure it includes water, water, and more water.

FitMe to Change the Way I "Wind Down"

So can I really change my habit of "winding down"? Is it really possible, after a long day of work plus the commute time, to actually bring myself to workout?

I asked all of my clients this question, and they pretty much all said the same thing about working out at the end of the day. None of them want to do it, but at the end of the workout they all say, "Now I feel great, I feel more energized, I feel like doing something better than vegging out in front of my TV."

As I have said before, doing what I do for such a long time, you get to meet all types of people—strong, self-motivated, lazy, ambitious, and more.

I give all the credit to my clients. When it comes to working out with me, the abilities they show and the achievements they have during the sessions are above and beyond amazing. I say that because there are only a few people that I know who really love working out. Sure, everyone loves the way they feel after, but not before. I remember a saying that another one of my clients used to tell me, "I love the thought of you coming over, I love the thought of what you have planned for the workout itself, I love the thought of the way my body will look, but what I really love most is not a thought. I love looking at your back the most, when you are leaving my place, that is when I love you the most." Can you believe it? It was like saying "Go away, and I will love you." Gee, what a job I've gotten myself into when every one of my clients "hate" me. Honestly, I don't really care.

So back to me giving credit for what one person can achieve by using a personal trainer. I remember one time I asked one of my clients, during a very hard workout, to stand on a Fit Ball; yes, you heard me right, stand on a Fit Ball (honestly, it was a joke, whoever has trained with me knows that I love making my sessions fun, where you can joke around while working very hard). He tried stepping on the Fit Ball, as if I had asked him to stand on a step.

He was about to stand on that ball so we could keep working out. What I am trying to say is that when it comes to working out with me or anyone of my trainers, it seems like the sky is not even close to the limit for my clients. Even if they complained about it they still did it, or at least tried their best to do it. When things get a bit rough, all they have to do is do the tasks I have given them.

You see, when you start working out, with or without a personal trainer, you must set your goals, long-term and short-term, just like any savings or investment account.

Sometimes, I'd meet clients who really wanted a personal trainer but couldn't find the time or couldn't afford the service for what their goals required. I used to give them tasks to do so that even if they could only afford to see a personal trainer once a week, they could still see the results they were aiming for.

If there is a performance issue with a client, either they book me for more times a week (out of the question of course 🙂) or I will help them with the task at hand. So I had to come up with a way for my clients to see that they can do it even if I am not around.

For the first week, I ask them to think of the moment that they get home from work, to visualize how it's going to look or maybe even visualize how it is going to be. How will they turn on the treadmill (if they have one) or whatever machine they are going to use? (Don't worry if you don't have a good machine at home, you don't need to run out and get one, you will be surprised what a good sofa and five minutes of commercial break can do for your legs). I ask them to visualize the moment when they enter their home and see themselves turning the machine on. Now, most of you are probably thinking about how hungry you are after being at work and sitting in traffic, and don't get me wrong, I do feel your concern, but first, we are talking about only five minutes. Later on in the book we will talk about your safety net. Now let's get back on track please.

Once we have that vision in our minds, firm and strong, we start with five minutes, only five minutes, and yes, even in your work clothing if you don't want to change, (although it would be best to change, wearing the right kind of clothing helps to get the mind into it.) Once your mind is set and you are on the first minute, I prepare my clients by letting them know that chances are they will want to do more once the five minutes are over, but I force them to stop once five minutes are up. And that is their task for the first week, only five minutes. I tell them that if they don't do the five minutes a day for the time scheduled, in the next session I will calculate the sum of five minutes times let's say six days, and during our next workout I will make them do a full thirty minutes, no breaks, and I'll just watch them on their treadmill, because it is all about making the habit a part of their new way of living.

The thing is that it doesn't make sense for them to pay a personal trainer to watch them while they walk since they know that I can get them to do much more than walking or jogging. Since they don't want to miss a workout they start to do the five minutes.

After the first week, I take it up to ten minutes. I tell them that it might be the opposite now; they might want to stop after seven or eight minutes, but they must stay strong and finish the ten minutes. I tell them that it is only their mind tricking them into thinking that they have something better to do. My dear friend, vegging out is not better, and if you think you do have something better, doing it ten minutes later will not kill you. Please don't tell me that your favourite TV show is on since you can watch it while you workout, or record it, or, and here's a cool fact, cutting your TV time by 50% can help you lose 100 calories a day. But if you must be in front of the TV, let's make a deal. For every show that you watch, you have to stand during every other commercial break. Remember, there are things you can do with a good sofa and five minutes of commercial break. Standing is one of them.

If they are having a week where they are very tired I tell them to go back to five minutes. However, every day I tell them to add two minutes to the regime until they are at twenty-five minutes. Basically after four weeks they will have adopted a gentle and elegant new habit of twenty-five minutes of activity at the end of the day.

Trust me, those twenty-five minutes will be your most precious time of the day. Once you start this habit, your mind will help you to dream again while you are sleeping, but you will dream with endorphins running through your blood. You might process some negative emotion like anger or stress through that activity. Hence, working out is a great way to change the habit of winding down to something more effective. It is the perfect time to clear your mind.

Summary:

First week – 5 minutes, NO MORE

Second week – 10 minutes, NO LESS and no more

Third week – go back to 5 minutes and increase 2 minutes every day until you reach 25 minutes

Tip: Since most people walk into the kitchen when they get home, I would suggest, if your spouse would not get angry, leaving your workout clothes in the kitchen or in a place where they will be the first thing you see. That way, when you walk into the kitchen, who knows, you might end up having a cup of water and changing your clothes.

FitMe is Opening a Calorie-Checking Account

Let's open a checking account for you. Sometimes I like to look at our daily and weekly calorie consumption as a checking account. I start the day with X amount of $ and I have to decide what I am going to spend or invest my money on or in.

Am I going to make investments, or am I going to spend it on nothing (or maybe I should say a moment of pleasure)? It's like when you're shopping and you buy something just because it was on sale, or because the colour was unique, or because you felt like it.

Well, it's the same thing with food. We start the day with a credit, which is X amount of calories that we need to get through the day (in general, and this is different for each of us, the average woman needs 1200 calories a day and the average man needs 1500 over a 24 hour period.) The kind of calories that we will consume is a choice that we make every time we consume something.

Sometimes we just take things for granted, but a moment of thinking about what you are about to eat can help you to save a lot of your calorie credit. Going back to the biggest question of all in one word: DIET = Do I Eat That? Just by asking this question, you are getting yourself to think about it.

So to continue with this metaphor, it is pretty obvious that good long-term investments are things like whole grains, veggies, etc. And the spending for a small amount of pleasure would be on things like sugar, salt, junk food, etc.

When you overspend your credit or go off your balance, you start paying interest. Interest is an annual or monthly charge, but it is being accumulated on a daily basis, we just pay it at the end of the month. If you fully pay off your interest then you might still be a little bit off-balance (like gaining one or two pounds, but it wouldn't really be noticeable), but if you keep failing to pay off what you spend it will accumulate until you are off-balance, and the cycle will keep going until you put a stop to it.

The same thing goes for your calories. You can consume them all in one meal and be responsible for the feeling it will give you, or you can spread them through small meals throughout the whole day. You can have them at night or during the day, as long as you make sure that you are giving your body what it needs and not your mind what it wishes to consume.

I am often asked how to avoid snacking while watching TV. Or how to avoid snacking in general. The obvious thing is to simply say "don't snack" or "don't watch TV," but the best thing I can say, and this always works for me, is that since we all know we can do only one thing at a time, the best thing to do is keep busy and just always be working. But I do understand that this is not easy. So if you can't keep yourself busy, and you can't stop snacking, let's make another deal. Let's agree that next time you are about to snack in front of the TV, consider how tired you are. Most people, when they are tired, tend to head for the kitchen instead of to bed. So what if it is only 10:00PM? You force your kids to go to bed early, tell them how important sleep is, worry about what they see versus what they hear. If you are honestly not tired then fine, as long as there are at least two hours before bedtime, go ahead, snack on your portion of almonds.

Another way to avoid eating or snacking is through another small commitment that you can make to yourself, and that is to make sure you eat only in the areas you have designated for eating in your home. I have a small eating area in my condo and I make sure to use it only for that. The second thing is that when I watch TV (which is really only on the weekend), I am only allowed to have water, tea or coffee. Eating in front of the TV is out of the question. I made that commitment to myself a long time ago. Try it! I'm telling you, if it worked for me, who knows, it might work for you.

I know some will say that it's ok to eat in front of the TV as long as you have a veggie or fruit snack or something else healthy, but FitMe is all about new habits. FitMe is about making things right, even if sometimes "right" is a bit out of your comfort zone. Remember, it is being in your comfort zone that got you to think about the change you are stepping into. By making this choice, you will start to think more than once before getting up to snack on something in front of the TV. So, as you can see, this book is all about making the right choice and sticking to it. Again, in this case the choice is not about not eating in front of the TV; the choice is about eating in your eating area and making sure that eating is the only thing you do there.

So the day is almost over, and you have just realized that you have over-consumed calories for the day, the next chapter will teach you how to realize when you have over-eaten. This is the perfect time to pay up. Saying "Tomorrow I will pay for what I have over-consumed" should not be an option. Your pay time should take place immediately.

Move yourself—take yourself on a long walk, a jog, anything that will increase your heartbeat. That is taking full responsibility for your actions by understanding that even your personal trainer can't make up for it. You are the only one who can do it, so pick up your butt and move!

As you get into the workout regime, your metabolism will get better, your energy levels will go up, and you might even find yourself happier.

Tip: When you come home from work, instead of putting on your pyjamas, change that habit and get into your running shoes, even if you are not planning to go out for a run. The way we dress has an enormous influence on the way we behave. Wearing your running shoes in the house after work can create a craving in your body to go out. Take your partner or take your kids with you. It will do wonders for your relationship.

Summarize your snacking habits into one commitment. Instead of promising yourself, "I will never eat in front of the TV again," let's try the FitMe way. Say to yourself, "I am committed to eating only in the designated eating area of my house."

FitMe My 30-Day Food Diary

Normally, when I start working with a new client, even before we meet for our consultation, the first thing that I ask them to do is a 5-day food diary. I ask them to be as detailed as possible, even to describe what they were feeling in those moments before they were about to eat.

The purpose of this is mainly for me to learn my client's lifestyle, since each and every person is different. When does their day begin and when does it end? How active is their day? Now, I must say that yes, it is annoying to walk around and write down every single thing that you eat, but most of my clients, before handing me their food diaries, will start to verbalize their daily eating habits, which is my favourite part. Most of them will give me a list of what they wished they ate, and if it's not a wish list, it's a list of what they are supposedly eating. They will give me some sort of information on how much they eat, and, while they lay out for me the healthy menu that they are so proud of, I often ask myself, "Heck, why do you need me if you eat the way you eat?" Obviously, I insist on receiving the five-day food diary, mostly so that my clients can get an understanding of where they are at. Most importantly, I always tell them not to try to make it look better than it is. "You already hired me, so you might as well be as honest as possible, not with me, but mainly with yourself." In most cases, once the five day period is over and they hand me their food diary, it is almost never anything close to what they have told me. It is not that they are lying, but the client will say to me, "I had no clue that this is what and how I actually eat."

You must understand that when I ask a new client to start a food diary, they must keep it with them 24/7 and anything that enters their mouth must be recorded on paper.

Quite often, people are shocked to realize that they didn't even notice how much they were about to eat. Most of them admitted that, as a result of keeping the food diary, there was more than one instance where they passed on eating one thing or another so that I wouldn't see how badly they were truly eating.

For me, that realization is the most important point of all. If this is the impact of keeping a 5-day food diary, what would the impact of keeping a 30-day FitMe food diary be? First of all, I will say that I now know the reason for doing it for 30 days. Normally, after five days, I would recommend a menu that aimed to balance my client's body needs along with their goals.

However, the difference between what I would recommend for them to eat and what they actually ate was huge. The difference was almost as big as the difference between their verbal food diary and the one they actually wrote.

That's when I realized that with some of my clients (and it doesn't mean they are necessarily less determined or less motivated, just that everyone is different), that I had to insist on them getting into the 30-day cycle. The 30-day cycle is a perfect match for your calorie-checking account. I make my clients a simple page with spaces to fill in, and once a week we get together to check how their week went. It was not about figuring out what they did wrong; it was about helping them to understand how they can do better for themselves, and where they stood in terms of their calorie-checking account. It was about letting them see that, just like any debt, once you start it, it just keeps growing.

Anyway, once we started to do things this way, things got much easier. My clients' self-awareness increased and they began to be more cautious about the choices they were making.

The end results, besides helping my clients to achieve their goals, were amazing because we managed to bring a new positive habit into their lives—self-awareness.

At the end of this book, I have re-created for you the same spreadsheet that I give to some of my clients so that you can start your own FitMe 30-day food diary. Even though you will be doing it yourself, it will be great when at the end of the week you are able to see how you ate. You will be able to determine where you could have chosen one thing versus the other, and to see that maybe this weekend you might need to be a bit more active in order to balance your checking account.

Tip: Ignore all of your excuses, because at the end of the day that's all they are, excuses.

Please allow me to share with you that when I started to write this book I was pumped to do so, mostly for my clients. I didn't think it would be published or spread very far, but I have to admit that as much as I was pumped to start writing the book, it took me exactly three days to think of all the reasons why I should stop. Anything that you can think of came to mind—who will want to read this book (even though I am writing it for my clients, why would they want to read it, they hear it from me almost three times a week)? Would anyone find it useful? I went on and on and on, which is how I came up with the tip at the end of this chapter. All I had to do was act in spite of the excuses that I gave myself. And hopefully I will be able to help even one person transform his or her life into one that is more balanced, healthier, and joyful.

FitMe to Become CEO

Are you kidding me? FitMe to become CEO? CEO of what?

Big changes require small steps. Often, people see me as someone who does not know how to enjoy life. How is it possible to live my life the way I do? Why would I even want to live like that? Some people call me ascetic, and to an extent they might be right.

However, I don't feel that way. I have no guilty feeling from day-to-day, and I can definitely say that I do not feel like I am missing something during the day. The people who know me are always hearing that I feel amazing, and since I have been on the other side of things, it is very easy for me to continue making the right choices for my body and mind. Now that I have been to both extremes, I can say that I am now the CEO of my body. What makes me CEO? As far as I know, CEOs are the ones who are calling all the shots in the operation, even after discussing it with all their assistants.

I must tell you that it wasn't always like that. It wasn't always as easy as it is now, and even now I don't know if easy is the right term to use, but until I come up with something better I guess I will use this one. But I do think that it took me a while to reset my mind. I think that only today can I finally say that I understand and have set my mind to a new way of living. What I am saying is that it was a long process to get to where I am today.

I was over 230 pounds, I was a smoker, I was a drinker, I was a clubber, you name it and I can proudly say that I have been there and done that. Making the transformation from where I was to where I am now required tons of effort and lots of patience. Maybe the best way to explain it is that it required lots of practice, and for the most part, this is how I try to get my clients to think. I avoid making them feel like crap for eating unhealthy things or not exercising, because I know that in most cases they have already given themselves a hard time. They have already gotten mad at themselves for making the same mistakes, but as I said, it is a matter of practice. It is not about how low you take yourself; it is about how quickly you push yourself forward again, and it's about how quickly you get yourself back on track.

You might wonder how come I am only giving you my personal story at the end of the book. I chose to tell you my own story at the end since I wanted you to remember that changing your life is a process, and that while you might be extremely pumped to start in the beginning, while you might have the urge to go through your whole kitchen and throw everything in the garbage and buy all healthy food, or run and sign up at your nearest gym, or even call FitMe Training and book your free consultation, it's important to remember that this is a process. Don't get me wrong, I am not trying to harm your motivation. My aim is to help you to be realistic. I am doing my best to help you to balance your motivation with your ambition. However, to make things a bit easier, there is a tip I can give you that, had I had it a long time ago, would have made things much easier for me.

As you may have noticed in some of the previous chapters, I use metaphors about life to describe almost anything involving food. Since food is a big part of my life it's easy for me to make these kinds of analogies.

So now I will take the whole "big picture" of living a healthy lifestyle and break it down. Each and every one of us is capable of leading a healthy lifestyle in one way or the other. Even for me, though some people tell me that I am too extreme (even my partner in life thinks that I tend to go too far), there are some who would say that I am far from being extreme.

If you look at any successful CEO of a company, a manager or really any business person, male or female, they all work with goals, both short- and long-term, and they all have big visions. So we need to be clear about our vision, and that is a vision for a healthy lifestyle.

The next step will be creating it, but first you need to envision it, create your own language with which to talk about it, using all the tools I have given you.

By now you should already have your 30-day food diary. This is a great starting point, since it is the tool you will use to decide which foods should be kept in your life and which ones you think should be replaced. Having your 30-day food diary, including the four reviews you had at the end of each week, can help to show you what is realistic to demand from yourself. You can always aim to reach the stars, but it's okay to reach the sky as well, as long as you try.

So once you have identified your weaknesses and strengths, I will ask you to once again keep a 30-day food diary, but this time you will choose up to three habits that you are going to change. And you are going to stick to those three habits only. There will be no adding or taking away, just like with the five to twenty-five minute jog.

So, for example, let's say that you have decided you can commit to drinking more water each day, drinking less coffee, and engaging in more activity.

For the next 30 days, commit yourself to drinking two cups of water first thing in the morning regardless of the amount of water you normally drink.

Cut your coffee consumption by 50%. Do the calculations— if you drink one cup a day and you wish to cut it out, drink half the cup and give away the rest.

Being more active does not necessarily mean going to the gym or exercising more. First of all, it is for you to decide what it means to be more active, but as far as I see it, even cleaning the house once a week by yourself instead of having your cleaning lady come over is a way to be more active. You could also take the stairs instead of the elevator or park far away from the entrance of the mall. Try to keep in mind the "good sofa" and the five-minute commercial break. Stand the whole time the commercials are on.

Assuming that this is your starting point, commit yourself to it by writing it down as your monthly task, and remember that you can only be a great self-manager once you begin to take action.

FitMe CEO: Be patient with yourself and give yourself credit when deserved.

FitMe to My 3-Breath "Prayer"

The 3-breath prayer, are we getting religious here? No, I am honestly not getting religious with you. However, breathing is a big part of my being, a big part of all human nature, and as a yoga teacher and breathing practitioner I understand all the benefits that proper breathing can offer you. I couldn't not include this chapter; I see it as a gift, one that you can choose to accept, or not.

I remember the first time I went to a yoga class. It was Ashtanga yoga, very high impact, very quick flow. I was already working out 6 times a week and in great shape, very fit. However, as I was doing my best to follow the teacher's instructions and to breathe as she was asking, I found that the hardest part of the class for me was breathing. From warrior to cobra to downward dog (yoga poses), I was unable to inhale and exhale correctly and do the motion at the same time. I felt like my breath was telling me to slow down, but the motion required me to move quickly. I knew that something was off, so I decided to continue the class and focus only on the poses themselves and let my body take care of the breathing. It is amazing how sometimes, when you do not think and just do, your body can make things happen for you. That was exactly what my body did. Some will say that I wasn't really doing yoga if I wasn't breathing while posing, and they may be right, but I did something much better. I gave my body the freedom to breathe, and I did my best to allow it to do so.

After leaving the class and trying to figure it out, I started to practice my breathing. I will often hear people say to one another "Just breathe," not knowing how difficult that can actually be. Even though it is something that you never stop doing, it is difficult to be aware of exactly how you're doing it. So again, trying to force my body to breathe deeply didn't work for me and I realized that it would require practice. So I started practising in another way. Instead of trying to breathe and making things harder for myself, I started to just be aware of my breath and find its flow. I was trying to listen to my body breathing and to count how many seconds it took me to exhale. Was I breathing from my chest, or my belly? I slowly began to analyze what was happening as I breathed, and just by doing that I have learned how to participate in breathing with my body, and how to gain control of the way I breathe, the sound of my breath, and how long I breathe for.

This change had a huge impact on the way I was working out at the gym. I slowly changed the way I lift weights, the way I sit, the way I sit while I drive, and today I can say that I have reached the point where no matter what I am doing I am doing my best to ensure that my body has the space it needs to breathe properly. Short breaths or long, the important thing is that the body has space to take them.

Tip: During high-impact workouts, allow yourself to breathe loudly, and ensure that you exhale at least as much as you inhale.

So what does breathing have to do with your new journey of creating a healthy lifestyle? You will be surprised at the impact that the 3-breath "prayer" can have on your self-awareness.

While learning to be an active participant in the way I breathe, I have committed myself to what I call the 3-breath "prayer." Don't worry, I am not trying to preach any religion whatsoever. I am giving you an amazing tool that will help you to actually practice all the chapters in this book.

So this was my commitment: For 30 days, before anything entered my mouth, even something like brushing my teeth or drinking a cup of water, I committed myself to stopping just beforehand and taking 3 inhales and 3 exhales. Not necessarily deep ones, but just 3 breaths. It had an amazing impact on my day-to-day activities and on my eating, because for someone who eats 5- 6 times a day not including drinking water, it turned out to be a lot of 3-breaths to count. I began to see things from a different perspective. Slowly I became more and more aware of what I was eating. I even found myself skipping snacks and having water instead because I would realize that I was only thirsty, not hungry.

Learning to practice my breathing has become a big part of my day-to-day life. If you wish to learn more about it I recommend the book *Light on Pranayama: The Yogic Art of Breathing* by B.K.S. Iyengar.

If I was asked to close this book with a single tip on top of everything else I have told you so far (and don't get me wrong, it's not that this tip is the most important one, they are all equally important), but for me this tip is just as precious as breathing is. My tip is this: do whatever you can think of in order to be fully aware of when it is that you are thirsty versus when it is that you are hungry. Most people don't really know how to tell the difference and will generally eat before drinking water, or if they don't eat they'll have coffee instead of water. Try to keep a bottle of water with you everywhere you go and sip it every hour or so. It will help you to stay in tune with whether your hunger is real or not.

FitMe Is Asking the Big Questions

So yes, I have given you all the great tools one can ask for, but is it going to be the answer? Is that going to make you content with your body for life? Almost, here is one more thing for you to do. Please take a moment to answer the following question. Remember that you are the only one who will read the answers, so please allow yourself to be honest, try to repeat the question to yourself each time you get an answer, the more honest you are with yourself the faster and easier it will be to get the results you dream of:

1. What is it that holds me back from achieving the body I am dreaming of?

2. What can I do or be to change it?

Let the journey to your LIFE CHANGE begin.

FitMe Vegan Fitness

Honestly, it is not about brainwashing you to become vegan.

I left this chapter for the end of the book, although when I think about it, maybe this chapter should have been either the very first one or the introduction. This chapter is about my own story and journey; it's my story as a believer in vegan fitness. I wanted to make sure that my readers would feel that this book truly is about making the right choices for themselves, reading all the chapters in my book but in the end practicing what works best for them. All I am saying is that I am doing my best to ensure that I give only recommendations, tips and advice. Vegan fitness is what I personally practice and it happens to work amazingly for me, and though I think it is important to share it, teach and train it, not even for one single moment would I think of saying "this is the only way."

I often found myself wondering about the timing of this book. What is it that is going on in my life right now that actually allowed me to get this book written?

I think that there is more than one reason or answer. For me, I think that I now truly feel, after a long search and many trials that I have found a way of living that works perfectly for me.

You see, as a teenager and as a kid I was very fat. As I have mentioned before, I was over 230 pounds. As though that wasn't enough, when I was 13 years old I started smoking, and at the age of 15 I added a little spice by beginning to drink alcohol (you can see where this is going.)

I must admit that even as a fat boy I was never bullied by my friends. I was maybe bullied a little bit by family, but with them it was out of concern. Though they didn't know how to help me they did the best with what they had. I was loved by my friends, which wasn't difficult to achieve. When you make everyone around you happy, then most people, if not everyone, will love you.

At the age of 16 or 17, I got sick for a week or two and everything I ate would make me throw up. As I always like to look at the positive side of anything in life, I noticed that I was losing weight. I liked that idea and continued to throw up, which got me on the path to bulimia and anorexia, a line I walked on for approximately three to five years. Thanks to a close friend who helped me every single day with my self-motivation (we are still friends today), I began to take my health into my own hands.

So yes, although I had lost all of the weight I wanted to while I was bulimic, the biggest fear that I had was of gaining it all back. Even when you are no longer bulimic there is a very long mental process you must go through to heal.

Today I can definitely say that I understand that life is just a process of growing up, of finding, of doing, of achieving, and of dreaming in your own way.

Looking back, I can see what an effect my sickness had on me, and yes I say sickness, because no matter how you look at it, bulimia, anorexia and all types of eating disorders are diseases.

Getting out of that phase of life drove me straight into the fitness world. I can't yet say health, since at that point it was still all about the results for me. There was a new struggle that I was facing; it was called the six-pack, and it was about developing a bulky, muscular body. That was my entrance into the fitness world. But again, that path has taught me the value of my body and has made my mind and body stronger.

So, you are asking, "Ok, but how is it that you decided that veganism and fitness belonged together?"

I will tell you how. In my experience and in that of my friends in the industry, there was always the same struggle. People have a tendency to go on a strict diet only in the 2 or 3 months leading up to summer to cut down some of their extra body fat percentage. You must remember that I am talking about people who are fit, take care of themselves, and already have low or average body fat. It is all about getting back their ab muscles (six-pack) during those 2 or 3 months. I used to go on a similar strict diet that for the most part was very similar to the first program a trainer would give an average trainee with no special needs. What I am trying to say is, that since it is difficult to keep with such a strict diet, most people only go on them once or twice a year.

Looking back, I had the feeling that something was missing. Yes, I felt great, yes, my body was healthy, but just like anything in life I wanted to aim for the best. I was trying to find that best and make it my own so that I could keep it with me all the time, so I wouldn't have to be strict with myself once or twice a year on a special diet. And then, about 14 years ago, I finally came across the vegan lifestyle.

I must admit that for me it started because I love animals, and until that day I had not really questioned where my food was coming from and what it contained aside from proteins.

Once I decided on a vegan lifestyle, all I could think about was the animals and not eating them. Yes, I was eating tofu and veggies, but something was missing, and slowly I began to feel that my body was lacking in energy. I felt that my physical performance during my workouts was also taking a beat-down.

Since giving up the vegan lifestyle was not an option, I began to learn more in-depth details about my body's needs. It was much harder, yes, but it really paid off.

Here is why: First of all, I was eating much more BUT felt lighter than ever. I had lost some of my body fat percentage without even intending to. I was more energized.

There are many other benefits that I could list here, but honestly I don't really want to brag. Even my muscle performance at the gym and in yoga was above and beyond normal. And that was how I got into vegan fitness.

So, what does vegan fitness mean? First, it means not eating chicken, meat, fish, dairy, or honey. It is about eating an abundance of fruits, veggies, nuts, grains and anything that comes from plants. It's about enzymes, minerals and vitamins, real nutrients, not just supplements.

It's about living a life where calories have almost no meaning, it's about constantly eating fresh and nourishing meals; it's about loving your body all the time since you love living in it.

For me, being able to write this book now after all the trials I have overcome in past years means knowing that I am finally content with my achievements, and that I am finally more than just satisfied with my body.

You might choose to become vegan, you might choose not to, but I did, and I am doing my best to share my way.

FitMe Certified Recipes

Breakfast or Snack Ideas

Banana "Cereal"

1/5 of a banana

1/2 an apple

1 tablespoon of raw sunflower seeds

1 teaspoon of raw sesame seeds

1 cup of silk almond milk/soy milk/rice milk

Instructions:

Place all the dry ingredients in a bowl. Add the cup of milk of your choice and bon appetite!

*Homemade Tofu Protein Shake

150 grams raw tofu

1/5 of a banana

3 dates

1 cup of water (you can also use almond milk or rice milk, however this will increase the level of sugar)

Instructions:

Place all the ingredients in blender and blend to desired texture.

Note: For chocolate flavour, you can add half a teaspoon of organic cocoa powder and a pinch of cinnamon (not a must)

*Homemade Veggie Protein Juice

2 cups of bean sprouts

2 celery sticks

½ a green apple

Instructions:

Place the green apple and celery in a juicer. Pour the juice into a food processor along with the bean sprouts and enjoy your protein shake.

*The proteins in the homemade juice come from the bean sprouts, so you can play around with the flavours of fruit and veggies that you are adding. In this case, because it is a breakfast shake, there is relatively high level of sugar from both the celery and apple.

Energy Meal Ideas

5-Coloured Quinoa Salad

½ green pepper

½ red pepper

½ yellow pepper

½ orange pepper

1 teaspoon black sesame seeds

1 cup of cooked Quinoa

1 teaspoon olive or flaxseed oil

The juice of 1 fully squeezed lemon

¼ cup of chopped dill and chopped mint

Instructions:

Take all 4 peppers and chop into tiny pieces. Place peppers in a salad bowl, add all other ingredients, and mix well. Add raw sunflower seeds to the top for decoration when serving.

Tofu Green Salad

100 grams of cubed tofu

2 tablespoons of cooked chickpeas

Mixed greens

1 very thinly sliced green apple

1 teaspoon of grape honey or date honey

1 teaspoon of olive oil

The juice of 1 fully squeezed lemon

Instructions:

Place tofu into a pan and grill until golden on all sides. Place mixed greens into a salad bowl and add the tofu. Add the apple, chickpeas, olive oil, lemon and grape syrup or silan (date honey.) Mix it all together, and bon appetite!

Green Millet Salad (can be served hot or cold)

1 cup cooked millet

½ cup chopped fennel

½ cup chopped zucchini

¼ cup chopped green olives

¼ cup chopped parsley

½ cup chopped celery

1 tablespoon olive oil

1 tablespoon flax seeds

Instructions:

Heat up the olive oil in a wok pan. Add the fennel, zucchini and celery, and wait for them to get just a bit soft (2-3 minutes.) Add the parsley and olives, mix well and give it another 2-3 minutes on the stove. Then add the cooked millet and the flax seeds. Stir gently but well, and serve to enjoy.

Note: Though the millet is relatively high in protein, if you still wish to boost it up, you can add 1 cup of chopped bean sprouts while stirring the fennel, celery and zucchini.

Spinach Tofu

150 grams of cubed tofu

Bunch of spinach leaves

1 chopped tomato

1 chopped clove of garlic

1 teaspoon of olive oil

Instructions:

Heat the olive oil in a pan (a wok pan is great, or any iron pan you like.) Once the oil is heated, add the cubes of tofu and fry them lightly. Add spinach, tomato and garlic. Serve once the spinach has softened. Sprinkle sesame seeds for garnish.

Note: this dish can be served with the green millet salad

Chipotle Tofu and Fennel

150 grams of cubed tofu

1 cup chopped fennel

½ cup chopped celery

½ cup green zucchini

½ teaspoon chipotle spice

1 teaspoon flaxseed oil or olive oil

Instructions:

Place tofu in a bowl with 1 teaspoon of oil (flax seeds or olive.) Mix together until fully blended. Start grilling on hot pan. Slowly add celery, fennel, and then zucchini. (Note: to keep the dish crunchy, try to add the zucchini only in the few last minutes.)

Sprinkle with sesame seeds and a bit of lemon, and then serve.

We Begin the Talk, You Begin the Journey

Do you want to lead a healthier life but don't know where to begin? Do you want to feel stronger, energized and more vital? *Dangerous Love* will help you to create a better life for yourself. This book will teach you how to:

- Manage your food cravings

- Make healthier food choices

- Learn how to balance your needs and wants

- Breathe properly

- Become a role model for your loved ones

- Eat a "jog meal"

- Motivate yourself to start exercising

- Open a calorie checking account

- Keep a food diary

- Become CEO of your own body

Together we will begin our journey to a healthier, better life.

Thank you for taking the time to read this book. I am wishing you lots of luck on your journey for a life change.

Call to book 30 days wellness coaching or to join one of Ilan's Life Change seminars by contacting FitMe Training head office:

Email: results@fitmetraining.com

Cell:1.647.216.7078

And remember we only help you to: *"Explore your strength. Discover your abilities."*

Made in the USA
Middletown, DE
26 October 2018